Practical Ethics for Students, Interns, and Residents

A Short Reference Manual

Third Edition

Charles Junkerman, M.D.
Professor Emeritus, Department of Medicine,
Center for the Study of Bioethics,
Medical College of Wisconsin

Arthur Derse, J.D., M.D.
Professor of Bioethics and Emergency Medicine,
Director for Medical and Legal Affairs,
Associate Director of the Center for the Study of Bioethics,
Medical College of Wisconsin

David Schiedermayer, M.D.
Hospitalist, Waukesha Memorial Hospital,
Waukesha, Wisconsin

For Anne, Deidre, and Kim,
practical ethicists in our lives, and for
Abraham Verghese, M.D., medical humanitarian

The authors and publisher have made every effort to ensure that the recommendations for actions, drugs, and doses set forth in this manual are in accord with current behavior and practice at the time of publication. However, in view of changing practice, physicians-in-training should consult with attending physicians at their own institutions if questions arise. Neither the authors nor the publisher are offering specific medical or legal advice.

University Publishing Group, Inc.
Hagerstown, Maryland 21740
1-800-654-8188
www.upgbooks.com

CONTENTS

INTRODUCTION

The concepts described here are as important to patient care as any diagnostic or management techniques. Evaluative strategies and therapeutic interventions will change frequently, but if the physician-in-training can master the art of communication with patients and can learn to identify and resolve ethical problems, he or she will have acquired enduring, career-enhancing skills.

This text contains a brief overview of the information needed to provide comprehensive, ethical, patient-centered care. Each section contains concise information on a topic. Many of the sections include additional material and a list of a few important references for those who wish to pursue further a given subject.

ACKNOWLEDGMENTS

Many residents in medicine and fellow faculty members at the Medical College of Wisconsin reviewed the text and provided valuable suggestions. The authors are especially appreciative of the encouragement offered by our editor, Ms. Leslie LeBlanc, and of her support for a short, physician-friendly ethics manual. The early assistance of Dr. Mahendr S. Kochar, Professor of Medicine and Senior Associate Dean for Graduate Medical Education, was invaluable. Review by Dr. Mark Adams, Dr. Carl Chan, Dr. Elsa Cohen, Dr. William Greaves, Dr. Robert Nelson, Dr. David Weissman, Ms. Sandy Pasch, and Attorney Robyn Shapiro has enhanced the accuracy of particular sections and is greatly appreciated. Dr. Rebekah Wang-Cheng supplied much of the text for the section on difficult patients. Thorough review and cogent comments by our colleagues — Dr. Dale Berg, Dr. John La Puma, and Dr. Kenneth Simpson — have resulted in a more readable text.

I. DO NOT RESUSCITATE (DNR)

DISCUSSION WITH THE PATIENT

The issue of cardiopulmonary resuscitation (CPR) should be addressed early in the treatment course of a patient with serious illness in whom cardiac or pulmonary arrest is likely. The subject should be approached sensitively as part of the overall therapeutic plan. The comfort and therapeutic measures that will remain in effect should be emphasized and discussed first.

AUTHORITY FOR DNR

Legal authority for the decision (in order of importance):
1. Request of a decisional patient (a patient who has decision-making capacity; see section IV)
2. Dictates of an advance directive
3. Judgment of guardian or healthcare agent appointed in an advance directive

In some states, surrogacy laws establish a hierarchy of authority; in others, there is moral authority but no legal authority for the following (if one to three above are not available):
4. Concurrence by first-order relatives (spouse, adult children, or parents who may best know the patient's wishes)
5. Opinions of other relatives or friends who are able to provide a "substituted judgment" (section IV, page 22) or who agree upon the best interest of the patient
6. If no relatives or friends are available for consultation, base the decision on medical indications and the best interest of the patient, taking into account whether CPR would further the reasonable personal medical goals of this particular patient.

WHAT THE DNR ORDER SHOULD INCLUDE

1. The order should be written by the attending physician or by a house officer at the request of the attending physician.
2. The progress notes should include documentation of:
    *   The medical indication for DNR or contraindication to CPR
    *   Advice of consultants (if any)
    *   Authority for the decision (see above discussion).
3. The order should include specific orders about what treatments are to continue. Specific orders should be in writing to avoid misunderstandings. Ordinarily, DNR simply means "no CPR." DNR may have no other significance and may be compatible with all other modalities of treatment including care in the intensive care unit. On the other hand, a DNR order may be the first step in the withdrawal of other treatment, in which case further clarification is necessary.

DNR ORDERS ON THE BASIS OF FUTILITY

In many institutions, a DNR order may be written on the basis of medical futility (see section IX, page 33). Another staff physician should concur in writing, and the justification for this judgment must be clearly indicated in the progress notes. Many policies stipulate that the patient or surrogate need not agree but must be notified. If the patient or surrogate disagrees with the decision, consultation with the institutional ethics committee is appropriate and hospital administration should be notified.

DISCUSSION WITH THE NURSING STAFF

The rationale and specific orders need to be discussed fully with the nursing staff and the patient's other caregivers so that there are no uncertainties about care plans. Patients are either DNR as clearly specified in the orders or they are full code. "Slow codes," "code grays," "show codes," or "Hollywood codes" are deceptive and place an unfair responsibility on the nursing service.

ATTENTION TO TLC

Many patients and their families fear abandonment when a DNR order is written, so it is important for physicians and nurses to be more attentive and aware of comfort measures. The patient and family must know from the outset that "no code" does not mean "no care."

ETHICS CONSULTATION

In the event that the authority for DNR is in question or a DNR order written on the basis of futility has created objections on the part of patient, family, or agent, an ethics consultation should be sought for clarification or mediation.

FURTHER READING

CPR was developed in the 1960s for treatment of sudden cardiac arrest in previously well individuals. Despite warnings that this technique could be inappropriate in other clinical situations, CPR became a default procedure. It was presumed that a patient wanted CPR unless there was a specific request to avoid it. This is a unique presumption in medicine.

Effectiveness of CPR

Public expectations of the success of CPR are quite unrealistic and do not match the statistics. Approximately 15 percent of hospitalized patients in whom resuscitation is attempted survive to discharge. Furthermore, numerous studies have reported virtually no survival to hospital discharge for patients with overwhelming pneumonia, renal failure, acute stroke, or multiple organ failure who have an in-hospital arrest. Patients over 70 years of age who have sepsis or metastatic carcinoma or whose resuscitation effort lasts more than 15 minutes are unlikely to survive. Recent research suggests, however, that CPR success varies from one institution to another and that the pre-arrest condition of the patient may be the most important predictor of success.

The best CPR results occur in persons who have a witnessed arrest on the basis of a ventricular dysrhythmia (not asystole) and who are successfully resuscitated within five minutes. CPR is successful in 25 percent of cardiac arrests that result from drug reaction or overdose. Extended CPR (more than 15 minutes) is reasonable in cases of subarachnoid hemorrhage, hypothermia, electric shock, and drug overdose.

Risks (burdens) of CPR
Of the patients who are successfully resuscitated, 25 to 50 percent have fractured ribs, fractured sternum, aspiration pneumonia, mediastinal hemorrhage, or pulmonary edema. Up to 10 percent of those whose CPR is successful may end up in a persistent vegetative state.

Discussion with the patient
When to talk about CPR with a patient is a matter of clinical judgment. For example, this discussion is probably unnecessary for a healthy woman entering the hospital in labor or a healthy young man coming in for a hernia repair. There is no need to unduly alarm such patients. Further, for such patients the desire for CPR and the prospect of a successful outcome can reasonably be presumed in the unlikely event of a catastrophe requiring resuscitation.

The discussion is mandatory, however, when patients are admitted for serious illnesses in which an arrest would not be unlikely or when patients have chronic illnesses and their condition may deteriorate. Unless previously expressed, the wishes of these patients cannot be presumed and, therefore, should be elicited.

Questions about the patient's desire for CPR need to be asked in the specific context of that patient's problems. One should avoid questions such as "Do you want us to do everything?" when "everything" is practically impossible for the patient or physician to define. Likewise, the question "Do you want us to start your heart if it stops?" implies falsely that such a result may be certain. The issue should be approached sensitively and as a part of the overall therapeutic program. The patient may need more information to make a decision. The physician should provide this information, along with some indication of whether CPR is recommended for this particular patient in this particular context. If the patient desires or the situation dictates, a more extensive discussion about the likely success and the burdens and risks of CPR should ensue.

If CPR would likely be futile (see section IX), a DNR order should follow a discussion emphasizing the positive measures that will be taken for the patient, the reassurance that the patient will not be abandoned, and the promise that all possible comfort measures will be provided. The physician can say that CPR is not a reasonable part of the patient's specific treatment "package." "We are not giving up on you; we are deciding against some treatment strategies that won't work and are not in your best interest."

Some ethicists advocate, with good reason, that DNR should be DNAR (do not attempt resuscitation) because DNR implies that a reasonable degree of success is possible. In patients for whom a DNR or no-CPR order is appropriate, the likelihood of success is usually minimal. To imply otherwise is to mislead the patient and thereby impair his or her autonomous judgment.

If some unforeseen event takes place in the hospital that makes cardiac or pulmonary arrest likely, the subject of code status should be brought up while the patient still has decision-making capacity (if possible). It is not ethical to wait purposefully until an acutely ill patient is no longer decisional in order to discuss code status with a surrogate.

Conflict between the patient's desire for "full code" and futility
The American Medical Association (AMA) Council on Judicial and Ethical Affairs has commented that resuscitative efforts "would be considered futile if they could not be expected to achieve the goals expressed by the informed patient. This definition of futility not only respects the autonomy and value judgments of individual patients but also allows for the professional judgment and guidance of physicians who render care to patients" (*JAMA.* 1991; 265:1868-1871).

Occasionally patients in whom CPR is certain to fail insist on the attempt. The physician is under no obligation to provide futile treatment. This right is recognized in law and ethics. Strategies for avoiding this conflict between the patient's desire for futile treatment and the physician's reluctance to use a treatment that is not medically indicated include the following:
1.   Avoid using the term *futility*, which is hard to define and even more difficult for patients to understand.

2. Determine the patient's goals in the present circumstances.
3. Determine in discussion with the patient or surrogate whether an attempt at resuscitation in light of its benefits and burdens will further these goals.

Relationship of DNR to advance directives (ADs)

DNR orders should not be confused with advance directives. ADs require interpretation and need to be incorporated into a treatment plan that includes specific orders consistent with the patient's wishes. This plan may or may not include a DNR order, but DNR is not usually a part of the AD (and normally shouldn't be, as the AD should express a patient's goals, and CPR may or may not help achieve those goals depending upon the medical circumstances). The existence of a living will usually indicates that a patient who has a terminal illness has considered forgoing CPR, but the existence of a power of attorney for healthcare does not necessarily imply the same intent.

DNR and the operating room (OR)

Anesthesiologists have expressed their discomfort with DNR orders in the OR because an arrest might occur during a procedure in the OR that is not related to the underlying disease, and this arrest may be easily managed with drugs. In this situation, anesthesiologists are reluctant to stand by and watch the patient die. Therefore, DNR policies should be modified so that ordinarily the DNR order is suspended when the patient goes to the OR (or undergoes a procedure such as cardiac catheterization) and is reinstituted automatically on discharge from the recovery room. The patient should be notified of the policy for placing the DNR order on hold and should have the option of overriding the policy, keeping the DNR order in effect through the procedure.

REFERENCES

American Medical Association, Council on Ethical and Judicial Affairs. Guidelines for appropriate use of do-not-resuscitate orders. *JAMA.* 1991;265:1868-1871.

Wenger NS, et al. Patients with DNR orders in the operating room: surgery, resuscitation, and outcomes. *J Clin Ethics.* 1997;8:250-257.

II. WITHDRAWAL OF TREATMENT

AUTHORITY FOR WITHDRAWAL OF TREATMENT
Authority for the decision (in order of importance):
1. Request of a decisional patient (section IV, page 20)
2. Dictates of an advance directive
3. Judgment of guardian or healthcare agent appointed in an advance directive
4. Approval of relatives (spouse, adult children, parents, adult siblings — in that order; order established by surrogate laws in some states and by convention in others)
5. Approval of close friends who know the patient's treatment preferences or are able to make decisions that promote the patient's best interest

DIFFERENCE BETWEEN WITHDRAWING AND WITHHOLDING
1. **Psychological difference**
   Psychologically, it is easier not to start a treatment than it is to stop it. But brief reflection demonstrates that this is illogical — the decision to omit treatment is just as much a willful judgment as the decision to withdraw it.
2. **"Up-front barrier"**
   When we decide not to start a specific treatment, we may be erecting an "up-front barrier" — that is, we may be denying in advance a treatment that might possibly be effective. Thus, a decision not to initiate treatment (to withhold treatment) must actually have stronger substantiating reasons than a decision to discontinue (withdraw) treatment that has clearly failed.
3. **Time-limited trial**
   When there is some uncertainty as to the effectiveness of a

treatment in furthering the patient's goals, the bias clearly must be in favor of a time-limited trial of treatment. If it later turns out to be ineffective and not beneficial for a particular patient in a given circumstance, the treatment can be stopped. By using this model, we have given the patient a reasonable chance of attaining the goals of a specific therapy.

WITHDRAWAL OF VENTILATORS

1. Patients with brain death

When the criteria for brain death have been satisfied (section VII, page 28), the person is legally dead, and there is no obligation to continue ventilation. The ventilator may be removed as soon as the pronouncement of death has been entered into the chart. Organ donation and sensitivity to the family's needs may legitimately delay this procedure for several hours.

2. Sentient patients

- **Method of withdrawal**

  When the decision has been made to remove a ventilator from a patient who is (or could be presumed to be) conscious and aware of the consequences, there is no good reason for weaning (the gradual decrease of ventilatory support), as the process often results in dyspnea and a sense of suffocation. After adequate sedation, the ventilator should be discontinued abruptly. Whether the endotracheal tube should be removed or remain in place for suctioning involves a judgment call.

- **Sedation**

  Before the ventilator is removed, the patient should be sedated heavily with a benzodiazepine or a barbiturate and morphine in doses adequate to produce unconsciousness but not sufficient to produce death. The sedation should be continued until death occurs. It requires the clinical judgment of the physician at the bedside to know how much and how long to sedate the patient in order to avoid further suffering.

- **Paralyzing agents**

  Under no circumstances should respiratory paralyzing agents be initiated during ventilator withdrawal because they hinder evaluation of the patient's suffering and discomfort. However, if a patient is already on these agents, it is not necessary to wait until they are entirely cleared from the system to begin the process of sedation and ventilator withdrawal.

WITHDRAWAL OF FLUID AND NUTRITION

1. **Patients in a persistent vegetative state (PVS)**

    In many states, advance directive statutes allow persons to state that they do not want fluid and nutrition if they are in a PVS (see section VIII, page 30). Such support can be withdrawn from these patients without causing suffering because, by definition, the symptoms of thirst and hunger are cortically mediated and cannot be present.

2. **Sentient patients**

    - **Decision to withdraw**

      In many states, power of attorney for healthcare laws specifically allow a person to give the agent the authority to withhold or to withdraw a feeding tube, regardless of whether the patient is in a PVS. The decisional patient, of course, retains the right to refuse artificially provided fluid and nutrition.

    - **Effect of withdrawal**

      When both food and fluid are withdrawn, death usually occurs from electrolyte imbalance and dehydration in 10 to 14 days. If fluid is maintained and food withdrawn, death occurs from starvation and may take many weeks. For this reason, both should be withdrawn or withheld. Patients are rarely uncomfortable in the clinical situations in which food and fluid are likely to be withdrawn. Ice chips and good oral care can assuage symptoms of dry mouth and provide comfort care.

- **Intravenous (IV) access**
Occasionally IV access is needed for palliative drug administration. A "keep-open" rate will not provide sufficient fluid to prolong the dying process significantly.

FURTHER READING

Rights of the decisional patient
The courts have made important statements on the rights of patients to decide about medical treatment. Justice B.N. Cardozo wrote in 1914, "Every human being of adult years and sound mind has a right to determine what shall be done with his own body" (Katz. 1972;526). The *Bartling* decision in California found, "Competent adult patients with serious illnesses which are probably incurable but have not been diagnosed as terminal have the right over the objections of their physicians and the hospital to have life support equipment disconnected despite the fact that withdrawal of such devices will surely hasten death."

Differences between medical treatment and supportive care
Important differences exist between medical treatment and supportive care. *Medical treatment* is provided by physicians and other health professionals; it is aimed at accomplishing the goals of medical practice. *Supportive care* can be provided by health professionals but is often provided by other caregivers such as family members; it is aimed at providing comfort to the dying patient. Providing human comfort is imperative, but no "technological im-

perative" exists. Thus, healthcare professionals are not obligated to provide specialized, life-sustaining treatment to every patient simply because such technology is available.

Difference between withdrawing and withholding
The President's Commission for the Study of Ethical Problems in Medicine and Biomedical and Behavioral Research noted in 1982 that the distinction between *withholding* (failing to initiate) therapy and *withdrawing* (discontinuing) therapy was not of moral importance. The commission believed that a justification adequate for not commencing a treatment was sufficient for ceasing a treatment that proved ineffective and noted that erecting a higher requirement for cessation might discourage trials of treatments that might sometimes be successful.

Right to withdrawal of fluid and nutrition
Some controversy has existed on whether administration of food and fluid through a feeding tube is a medical treatment or "ordinary care." This was effectively settled by two court decisions. In the New Jersey *Conroy* decision (1985), the court acknowledged the emotional significance of food but noted that feeding by implanted tubes is a medical procedure with inherent risks and possible side-effects, instituted by skilled careproviders to compensate for impaired physical functioning. The court said this procedure, analytically, is equivalent to artificial breathing using a respirator.

In an opinion in the U.S. Supreme Court *Cruzan* case (1990), Justice Sandra Day O'Connor said, "Artificial feeding cannot readily be distinguished from other forms of medical treatment. The techniques used to pass food and water into the patient's alimentary tract all involve some degree of intrusion and restraint. Requiring a competent adult to endure such procedures against her will burdens the patient's liberty, dignity and freedom to determine the course of her own treatment."

Effect of withdrawal of fluid and nutrition
Hypernatremia and hypercalcemia occur in many patients after withdrawal of fluid and nutrition. These changes, along with hyperosmolarity, azotemia, and increased endogenous opioids, often produce a sedative effect on the brain during the dying process. Hospice workers have provided other observations:

15

1. Persons near death often voluntarily stop eating and drinking and do not tolerate substantial volumes of enteral feedings.
2. Dying persons who are given "normal" replacement fluids commonly show signs of fluid overload, including distressing pulmonary edema.
3. Despite substantial physiological deficits, hospice patients almost never report feeling hunger or thirst. Dry mouth and lips are easily remedied by lubricants and ice chips.
4. Dehydration results in less vomiting and diarrhea, less need to suction secretions, and less dyspnea and peripheral edema.

REFERENCES

ACCP/SCCM Consensus Panel. Ethical and moral guidelines for the initiation, continuation, and withdrawal of intensive care. *Chest*. 1990;97:949-958.

American Medical Association, Council on Ethical and Judicial Affairs. Decisions near the end of life. *JAMA*. 1992;267:2229-2233.

American Thoracic Society. Withholding and withdrawing life-sustaining therapy. *Ann Intern Med*. 1991;115:478-484.

Bartling v. Superior Court. 209 CalRptr 220;163 Cal App 3d(1986).

Brody H, Campbell ML, Faber-Langendoen K, Ogle KS. Withdrawing intensive life-sustaining treatments: recommendations for a compassionate clinical management. *N Engl J Med*. 1997;336:652-657.

Conroy, In re. 98 N.J. 321, 486 A.2d 1209 (N.J. 1985).

Cruzan v. Missouri Dept of Health. 497 US; 111 LEd 2d 224, 110 SCt 2841 (1990).

Katz J. *Experimentation with Human Beings*. New York: Russell Sage Foundation; 1972.

Meisel A. Legal myths about terminating life support. *Arch Intern Med*. 1991;151:1497-1502.

President's Commission for the Study of Ethical Problems in Medicine and Biomedical and Behavioral Research. *Deciding to Forego Life-Sustaining Treatment: Ethical, Medical and Legal Issues in Treatment Decisions*. Washington, DC: US Government Printing Office; 1983.

III. INFORMED CONSENT

PURPOSE

The purpose of informed consent is to provide the patient with all of the information necessary to allow a person to make a prudent treatment choice on his or her own behalf.

ADEQUACY OF INFORMATION

According to the President's Commission for the Study of Ethical Problems in Medicine and Biomedical and Behavioral Research, adequate informed consent requires effort on the part of the physician to ensure comprehension; it involves far more than just a signature on the bottom of a list of possible complications. Such compilations can be so overwhelming that patients are unable to appreciate the truly significant information and to make sound decisions.

ELEMENTS OF INFORMED CONSENT

1. **Information**

   The patient must have a clear understanding of:
   - The disease process (diagnosis in understandable terms)
   - Prognosis
   - Benefits and burdens of recommended treatment
   - Benefits and burdens of reasonable alternative treatments
   - The likely effect of no treatment (this is always an option)

2. **Consent**

   Consent is the patient's voluntary, autonomous authorization to proceed with the proposed intervention.

OBTAINING INFORMED CONSENT

Informed consent always involves the following elements:
1. Adequate disclosure of information
2. Decisional capacity of the patient
3. Patient's comprehension of the information
4. Voluntariness (freedom from coercion)
5. Consent of the patient

DISCLOSURE STANDARDS USED BY THE COURTS

1. **Professional community standard**

   What a capable and reasonable medical practitioner in the same field would reveal to a patient under the same or similar circumstances (some states use this standard).

2. **Reasonable patient standard**

   Because of the recognition of patients' autonomy, another standard has been developed, which asks for the information that a reasonable patient would consider material to the decision of whether to consent to the procedure offered (the majority of states use this standard).

EXCEPTIONS TO THE INFORMED CONSENT REQUIREMENT

1. **Emergency privilege**
   - The patient must be unconscious, or without the capacity to make a decision, while no one legally authorized to act as agent for the patient is available.
   - Time must be of the essence, in the sense that there is a risk of serious bodily injury or death.
   - Under the circumstances, a reasonable person would consent.

2. Therapeutic privilege: disclosure would have an adverse effect on the patient's health
- The physician must take into account the circumstances of the patient.
- The physician must believe that a full disclosure of the information will have a significantly adverse impact on the patient. (This standard has been much abused in the past; it should be used infrequently and with great discretion.)

3. Patient does not have decisional capacity
The patient must be decisional for consent to be informed or free.

4. Waiver of rights
The patient does not desire to have information. The physician should not force the issue but should document it well and ask for permission to inform a surrogate.

REFERENCES

Brody H. Transparency: informed consent in primary care. *Hastings Cent Rep.* 1989;19(5):5-9.

Meisel A, Kuczewski M. Legal and ethical myths about informed consent. *Arch Intern Med.* 1996;156:2521-2526.

President's Commission for the Study of Ethical Problems in Medicine and Biomedical and Behavioral Research. *Making Health Care Decisions: The Ethical and Legal Implications of Informed Consent in the Patient-Physician Relationship.* Washington, DC: US Government Printing Office; 1982.

IV. COMPETENCE AND DECISION-MAKING CAPACITY

DEFINITIONS

1. **Competence**

   Competence and *incompetence* are legal terms that refer to the ability of a person to make decisions about his or her affairs. Technically, an adult patient remains legally competent until a court says otherwise.

2. **Decision-making capacity**

   Decision-making capacity is a medical term referring to an individual's ability to make medical decisions. Determination of decision-making capacity can be made by medical personnel and does not require a court hearing.

CLINICAL ASSESSMENT OF DECISION-MAKING CAPACITY

In assessing a patient's ability to make autonomous judgments, one must evaluate the three distinct aspects of decision-making capacity:

1. **Ability to understand**
   - The ability to comprehend the given information about diagnosis and treatment and to identify the issue at hand. (To test this, ask the patient to paraphrase the discussion.)
   - The ability to appreciate the impact of the disease and its consequences. (To test this, ask the patient to state the major options and the most likely outcome for each option.)

2. **Ability to evaluate**
   - The ability to deliberate in accordance with one's own values.

- The ability to manipulate information rationally and to compare risks and benefits of the options.
- The ability to make choices that are not irrational and to give the reasons for them.
- The ability to maintain a consistent choice over time.

3. Ability to communicate
- The ability to communicate choices. (To test this, ask the patient to state his or her choice of treatment options.)

If the patient demonstrates satisfactory responses in all three areas, he or she is said to have "decision-making capacity," to be "decisional," or to be "capacitated."

DEGREE OF CONFIDENCE IN A PATIENT'S DECISION-MAKING CAPACITY

1. If there is a favorable expectation from the patient's choice (little risk, large benefit), then a relatively low level of decision-making capacity is required.
2. If there is a balance of risk and benefit from the patient's choice, then a moderate level of decision-making capacity is required.
3. If expectations from the patient's choice are not favorable (great risk with little chance of benefit), then a high level of decision-making capacity is necessary.

THE MATURE MINOR

By legal definition, minors (under the age of 18 in most states) are not competent to make major healthcare decisions. Many states give minors limited autonomy; they may be allowed to obtain contraception, abortion, and treatment for venereal disease or substance abuse without parental permission. In many states, minors who are married or living independently and supporting themselves are considered to be "emancipated minors" and competent to make their own healthcare decisions. Moreover, developing case law on the "mature minor" now recognizes that as the adolescent's age increases toward maturity, he or she should have a progressively greater part in the decision-making process.

DECISION MAKING FOR INCAPACITATED PATIENTS

When a surrogate acts for an incapacitated patient, the basis for decision is one of the following:

1. Substituted judgment

This is the guideline the surrogate uses if the patient has expressed a preference before becoming incapacitated, or if the surrogate knows the patient well enough to determine what the patient would choose if he or she were still decisional.

2. Best interests

This is the standard the surrogate must use when he or she has no clear idea of what the patient might choose. It is what a reasonable person might choose in the same context and is based on what is ultimately best for this particular patient in these particular circumstances.

When a patient has a legal guardian, this individual has the right to refuse life-sustaining treatment based on the patient's best interests in the light of the diagnosis, prognosis, and medical goals of treatment.

DIFFICULTIES IN MAKING JUDGMENTS FOR THE INCAPACITATED PATIENT

There are several complications in making ethical decisions that are in the best interest of an incapacitated patient.

1. We do not know the wishes of the patient in regard to the withdrawal of life-sustaining treatment in the context of the immediate clinical situation.
2. Since we do not have the autonomous wishes of the incompetent patient to act upon, we must rely on surrogates and professionals to make these decisions.
3. It is preferable to make quality-of-life judgments based on the patient's own assessment. Because incompetent patients cannot provide this information, quality-of-life determinations become subjective on the part of others — a risky evaluation at best.

REFERENCES

Cohen LM, McCue JD, Green GM. Do clinical and formal assessments of the capacity of patients in the intensive care unit to make decisions agree? *Arch Intern Med.* 1993;153:2481-2485.

Miles SH, Koepp R, Weber EP. Advance end-of-life treatment planning. *Arch Intern Med.* 1996;156:1062-1068.

V. CONFIDENTIALITY

Patients' confidence that information given to a physician will remain private is an important element in the doctor-patient encounter. Without such assurance, patients might be unwilling to divulge information critical to their care. A physician's duty of confidentiality is reinforced by federal and state laws that restrict disclosure of information given by patients to their physicians. The federal Health Insurance Portability and Accountability Act (HIPAA) generally requires patient permission for disclosure to others, although patient consent is not required to disclose personal health information for purposes of treatment, payment, and healthcare operations.

BASIS FOR THE PRINCIPLE
1. Inherent respect for an individual's privacy and autonomy
2. Special trust relationship in the doctor-patient encounter
3. Element of promise in the Hippocratic Oath
4. The good of society
5. Prevention of harm to the patient.

EXCEPTIONS
There may be legal exceptions to the maintenance of confidentiality that necessitate divulgence. Among these are:
1. Testifying in court
2. Reporting communicable disease
3. Reporting child abuse, spouse abuse, or elder abuse
4. Reporting gunshot or suspicious wounds if there is a reasonable cause to believe they are the a result of a crime
5. Reporting for workers' compensation cases.

BREACH OF CONFIDENTIALITY

There may be situations in which there is an ethical demand for the physician to consider breaching patient confidentiality. Such a problem may occur when a patient who is HIV positive refuses to tell a sexual partner of the infection, placing the other at risk. The physician who is aware of this is in a bind between duty to the patient and the stronger ethical demand to warn an unsuspecting person of significant danger. Such a breach is justified when all of the following conditions apply:

1. A high probability exists of serious physical harm to an identifiable person
2. A likely benefit will result from breaking the confidence (for example, the harm can be prevented)
3. The breach is a last resort; persuasion and other approaches have failed
4. The breach is generalizable; it would be reasonable for a doctor to breach your confidence and to treat you in the same way if you were the patient.

Note: HIPAA provides exceptions to the requirement for patient consent for disclosures that are legally required. Examples include judicial or administrative proceedings; required reporting of abuse, neglect, or domestic violence; public health purposes; research; and worker's compensation proceedings.

REFERENCES

Brennan TA. AIDS and the limits of confidentiality: the physician's duty to warn contacts of seropositive individuals. *J Gen Intern Med.* 1989;4:242-246.

Gostin LO, et al. Privacy and security of personal information in a new health care system. *JAMA*. 1993;270:2487-2493.

Health and Public Policy Committee of the American College of Physicians and Infectious Diseases Society of America. Acquired immunodeficiency syndrome. *Ann Intern Med*. 1986;104:575-581.

HIPAA. 45 CFR Parts 160 and 164. December 28, 2000 as amended: May 31, 2002, August 14, 2002, February 20, 2003, and April 17, 2003.

VI. HEART-LUNG DEATH

The centuries-old determination of death is the heart-lung standard. All 50 states recognize heart-lung death — the cessation of heartbeat and respirations — as death.

STEPS IN PRONOUNCING DEATH
When called to pronounce a patient dead, observe the following steps:
1. Ascertain code status.
2. Check for hypothermia or drug overdose, which can be confounding factors.
3. Auscultate for respirations and heart tones.
4. Check corneal reflexes with a wisp of cotton or tissue.

The patient is pronounced dead if no positive responses are found to any of the above. Document the time of death in the chart.

VII. BRAIN DEATH

By definition, "whole brain" death occurs when the entire brain — including the cerebral cortex and the brain stem — has died. This definition of death has been endorsed by the American Medical Association and the American Bar Association. All 50 states recognize brain death, either by statute or through common law.

CRITERIA FOR DIAGNOSIS
1. A neurologic event adequate to produce brain death
2. Reliable examination showing absence of brain stem function

FINDINGS ON PHYSICAL EXAMINATION
1. Profound coma — "eyes-closed unconsciousness"
2. No eye movement; no pupillary response
3. No corneal reflexes
4. No cough or gag reflex; no motor response to pain
5. No spontaneous respiratory attempts off the ventilator. (There are several ways of testing for apnea. If the patient is a potential organ donor, this test should only be done after consultation with the transplant coordinator.)

LABORATORY CONFIRMATION
1. Radionuclide tracer shows no cerebral blood flow
2. Electroencephalogram (EEG) is not reliable, especially in cases of drug overdose or hypothermia.

LEGAL ASPECTS
If above criteria are satisfied, the patient is legally dead, and no further treatment is necessary. New York and New Jersey

allow certain exceptions to the declaration of brain death to accommodate personal religious beliefs.

It is important to document the time of death in the chart before turning off the ventilator.

HUMANITARIAN ASPECTS

Patients who are brain dead may not *look* dead. It is important to work with the family to help them acknowledge the death of their loved one. Occasionally, the ventilator needs to be left on for a slightly longer period to allow for this adjustment.

CONTROVERSIES

There is some current controversy about whether patients with cerebral cortical function loss but with a functioning brain stem (see section VIII on persistent vegetative state) should be included in an expanded definition of brain death. See also criteria of death in organ donation (section XIII).

REFERENCE

Halevy A, Brody B. Brain death: reconciling definitions, criteria, and tests. *Ann Intern Med.* 1993;119:519-525.

VIII. PERSISTENT VEGETATIVE STATE (PVS)

DEFINITION
Total loss of cerebral cortical function with a functioning brain stem.

CHARACTERISTICS OF PVS
1. Sleep-like coma for a few days to a few weeks. Then the eyes open, and sleep-wake cycles begin.
2. "Eyes-open unconsciousness." Eyes move in random fashion but do not focus or follow. Patient is "awake but unaware." (In cases other than PVS, when recovery does occur, true tracking of objects by the eyes is often the first sign of recovery. This must be differentiated from a brief turning of the eyes of the PVS patient toward the source of sound, which is a primitive reflex.)
3. Unintelligible grunts, screams; grimacing and chewing without purpose. Swallowing is uncoordinated, so the patient must be tube fed.
4. Many reflexes are present including corneal, cough, gag, and startle.
5. The presence of gross involuntary reflexive movement without purpose.

PROGNOSIS
After three months, prognosis for recovery is virtually nil. It may be possible to establish lack of recovery of independent function after 1 month in patients with PVS caused by cerebral hypoxia.

DIAGNOSIS

The diagnosis is clinical; no definitive laboratory test is available. Neurological consultation should be obtained for confirmation. PVS is not recognized in law as "death."

MANAGEMENT

1. Good communication is required to help family understand that the patient, by definition, cannot be suffering. Sensations such as pain, hunger, thirst, suffering — and joy and awareness — are cortically mediated and absent in PVS.
2. Usually the patient is not ventilator dependent, so the decision is whether to withdraw fluid and nutrition. This determination is easier to make if a patient has an advance directive or a reliable, informed surrogate decision maker.

FURTHER READING

Prognosis of PVS

One study reported that, following cerebral hypoxia-ischemia (the most common cause of PVS), no patient who remained vegetative for more than one month ever regained consciousness (*JAMA*. 1985;253:1420-1426). Some states require a period of three months in PVS for definitive diagnosis. The prognosis depends on the circumstances; in young adults and in cases of subarachnoid hemorrhage, it may take longer to predict the inability to recover independent function. The general rules to establish a "hopeless" prognosis are:
- three months after hypoxic episode in child or young adult
- 12 months after head injury in a child
- 6 months after head injury in an adult.

After these intervals, recovery is extremely unlikely and those few who recover remain nursing home patients with severe neurologic deficit, including the "locked-in" syndrome.

Prognosis in the coma phase following hypoxic-ischemic brain injury

Patients who will not regain independent function have these characteristics:
1. No pupillary light reflexes at time of initial exam

2. Lack corneal reflexes after the first day
3. Persistence of coma at seven days

The absence of oculocephalic reflexes or the absence of purposeful motor response to pain portend a poor prognosis.

Laboratory studies in PVS

Although there are no definitive studies, positron emission tomography (PET) scans of PVS patients have shown cortical glucose consumption to be at the same low level as that of patients in deep anesthesia. Serial computed tomography (CT) scans show significant and progressive atrophy but no specific changes. Autopsy studies routinely show bilateral hemispheric damage to a degree that is incompatible with consciousness.

Differentiation from "locked-in syndrome" and minimally conscious state

PVS must be differentiated from the "locked-in syndrome," in which patients are fully conscious but are quadriplegic and can only communicate through eye movements and blinking. PVS must also be differentiated from another subgroup of patients with severe and persistent alterations in consciousness who demonstrate inconsistent but discernible evidence of consciousness, such as the ability to localize sound and tactile stimuli and may have sustained visual fixation and pursuit. Nonetheless, prognosis for recovery in patients in a minimally conscious state (MCS) is extremely poor.

REFERENCES

American Medical Association, Council on Scientific Affairs and Council on Ethical and Judicial Affairs. Persistent vegetative state and the decision to withdraw or withhold life support. *JAMA*. 1990;263:426-430.

Cranford RE. The persistent vegetative state: the medical reality (getting the facts straight). *Hastings Cent Rep*. 1988;18:27-32.

Fins JJ, Schiff ND, Foley KM. Late recovery from the minimally conscious state: Ethical and policy implications. *Neurology*. 2007;68:304-307.

Giacino JT, Ashwal S, Childs N, et al. The minimally conscious state: definition and diagnostic criteria. *Neurology*.
2002;58:349-353.

Levy DE, et al. Predicting outcome from hypoxic ischemic coma. *JAMA*. 1985;253:1420-1426.

IX. FUTILITY/UNREASONABLE PATIENT REQUESTS

Sometimes patients make unreasonable requests: e.g., a computed tomography (CT) scan for tension headache or antibiotics for viral infection. Ethical principles support a physician's refusal to accede to a patient's demands to provide medical interventions that have no potential benefit or scientific merit — i.e., those that are futile.

FUTILITY

Futility is difficult to define, but the this definition seems reasonable: "Medical futility means any effort to provide a benefit to a patient that is highly likely to fail and whose rare exceptions cannot systematically be reproduced" (Schneiderman and Jecker.1995;11). Many ethicists believe that a distinction must be made between an *effect* that is limited to some part of the patient's body and the *benefit* that the patient has the capacity to appreciate and that improves the patient as a whole. For example, a ventilator that is effective in sustaining respiration may not be considered a benefit by a patient whose death from metastatic malignancy is imminent. Non-sentient patients (such as patients in a persistent vegetative state) cannot personally experience any intervention as a benefit. The term *futility* refers to a specific medical intervention applied to a specific patient at a particular time. The term does not refer to a general situation of treatment or to a patient personally.

REASONS FOR REQUESTS FOR FUTILE OR IRRATIONAL THERAPY

1. **Unrealistic goals of the patient and/or family**
   Physicians may fail to discuss achievable goals with the

patient in terms of the change that would most likely result from the specific intervention being considered.

2. **Guilt**
   Families may worry about betrayal of patient trust if they agree to withdrawal of treatment. They may also be compensating for past neglect or inattention.

3. **Confusion in formulation of the therapeutic plan**
   This situation is most likely to occur in serious illness with multiple consultants (and no one apparently in charge).

4. **Mistrust of physicians by the patient or family**
   Involvement of the primary care physician who knows the patient well may resolve this.

5. **Ethnic and socioeconomic differences**
   Poor patients may worry that any curtailment of services is rationing. Minority patients may be concerned about undertreatment as a form of discrimination.

6. **Denial mechanisms of the patient or family**
   The patient or family may refuse to come to terms with reliable information of a patient's impending death.

7. **Misunderstandings/language barriers**
   If an interpreter is necessary, he or she should be an objective observer, preferably with some medical translation training — not a family member.

8. **Religious issues**
   Family is awaiting or certain of a miraculous cure.

RIGHTS OF PATIENTS

1. **Negative rights (the right of refusal)**
   These are strong rights that include the right of a decisional patient to refuse any and all treatment. These rights are based on liberty and privacy. Physicians are obligated to respect such refusals.

2. Positive rights (the right to request a specific treatment)
These rights are weaker because they impose an obligation on others. Patients cannot demand treatment that is considered futile by the physician because this would obligate the physician to violate his/her professional integrity in order to provide the useless treatment.

GROUNDS FOR REFUSAL OF AN UNREASONABLE REQUEST
A doctor may refuse a patient's request for these reasons:
1. Request is for something outside the scope of good medical care. This judgment is based on lack of objective evidence for the effectiveness of the requested intervention.
2. Request requires the doctor to act illegally.
3. Request requires the doctor to violate a personal and professional standard of responsible medical practice.
4. Requested treatment cannot be anticipated to produce any beneficial result for this patient.

ADDITIONAL CAVEATS
1. When the request is for treatment that has reasonable potential for both benefit and harm, the preference of the fully informed patient must take precedence.
2. Decisions should not be made solely on the basis of economic considerations.
3. Usually when a physician decides not to comply with a patient's request, an opportunity for a second opinion should be offered.

ETHICAL CONCERNS
1. "The right of the patient to choose does not imply the right to demand care beyond appropriate options based on medi-

cal judgment and accepted standards of care, nor are physicians required to provide care in ways that in their personal judgment violate the principles of medical ethics" (*JAMA*. 1992;268:2282-2288).

2. "The well being principle circumscribes the range of alternatives offered to patients: informed consent does not mean that patients can insist upon anything they might want. Rather, it is a choice among medically accepted and available options, all of which are believed to have some possibility of promoting the patient's welfare" (President's Commission for the Study of Ethical Problems in Medicine and Biomedical and Behavioral Research. 1982:42-44).

LEGAL CONCERNS

The law does not outline standards for clinicians to use in deciding when to refuse unreasonable requests by patients. Rather, the law articulates general duties that arise from the doctor-patient relationship and its ethical framework. The courts, through the laws of professional negligence, enforce these duties, maintaining that failure to fulfill them may result in compensable harm to patients. The physician's primary legal duty is to possess and apply the knowledge and use the skill and care that is ordinarily used by reasonably well-qualified doctors in similar circumstances. This does not mean that the doctor must acquiesce to patients' demands that are unreasonable.

Many physicians unreasonably fear liability for not "doing everything," such as instituting every available technology when a patient requests it. The law rarely dictates the particulars of clinical practice and does not require that physicians do everything requested by a patient, agent, or guardian.

DIFFERENCE BETWEEN FUTILITY AND RATIONING

There is a danger that "futility" may be used as an excuse for decisions made on the basis of economic considerations — a real danger in a medical system driven by market forces.

It is particularly important to distinguish *futility* — a concept applied to a given patient and implying no apparent therapeutic benefit in that specific situation regardless of cost — from *rationing* — a concept that applies not to the individual but to society at large. Rationing also differs from futility in that it may acknowledge therapeutic benefit but deny it to some or all members of society because of cost.

THE CLINICIAN'S RESPONSE TO FUTILE SITUATIONS

It may be best to avoid the term *futility* in discussion with patients. One might instead use phrases such as "this won't help," or "this might even cause more problems." It is often better to approach discussions with patients in ways that will answer three questions:

1. What are the realistic goals of this particular patient in these particular circumstances?
2. Is the treatment being considered likely to achieve these goals without undue burden?
3. Is the planned intervention consistent with good medical practice.

Many requests for futile interventions result from incomplete or inadequate information. By spending time in careful communication with the patient (or surrogate) about reasonable expectations, the physician may avoid later confrontations. According to Paris: "If, after the physician has listened to the concern of family members (or the decisional patient) and explored the possibilities with them — including transfer of the patient to a willing physician — the family (or the decisional patient) persists in demands for continued life-prolonging treatment that the physician believes to be beyond well established medical criteria, the physician ought not to feel obliged to provide it. The physician's response in such cases should be: 'I'm sorry, but we don't do that here.' This is done not because the patient no longer has any value or because the physician lacks respect for the family's wishes. It is done because the obligation of physicians, as articulated in the Hippocratic oath, is to act for the benefit of the patient according to their ability and judgment." (*Cambridge Q*. 1993;2:147-149).

REFERENCES

American Medical Association, Council on Ethical and Judicial Affairs. Guidelines for CPR: ethical considerations in resuscitation. *JAMA*. 1992;268:2282-2288.

Loewy EH, Carlson RA. Futility and its wider implications. *Arch Intern Med*. 1993;153:429-431.

Paris JJ. Pipes, colanders, and leaky buckets: reflections on the futility debate. *Cambridge Q*. 1993;2:147-149.

President's Commission for the Study of Ethical Problems in Medicine and Biomedical and Behavioral Research. *Making Health Care Decisions: The Ethical and Legal Implications of Informed Consent in the Patient-Physician Relationship*. Washington, DC: US Government Printing Office; 1982:42-44.

Schneiderman LJ, Jecker NS. Is the treatment beneficial, experimental or futile? *Cambridge Q*. 1996;5:248-256.

Schneiderman LJ, Jecker NS. *Wrong Medicine*. Baltimore, Md: Johns Hopkins University Press; 1995.

Wear S, Logue G. The problem of medically futile treatment: falling back on a preventive ethics approach. *J Clin Ethics*. 1995;6:138-148.

X. THE DIFFICULT PATIENT

Some patients are very difficult to care for in a professional manner. They may engender feelings of anger, rejection, frustration, or resentment on the part of the physician. Taking care of such patients requires specific skills.

SPECIFIC SITUATIONS
1. **The seductive patient**

   Physician response: At first naivete, then confusion and embarrassment.

   Management tips:
   1. Always have another person present, especially for pelvic or genital exams.
   2. Be wary of accepting gifts.
   3. Be suspicious of frequent phone calls, especially after hours.
   4. Terminate relationship if necessary.

2. **The chronic somatizer**

   Physician response: Initially impatience, later rejection.

   Management tips:
   1. Establish a long-term, "one-doctor" relationship.
   2. Schedule frequent (every six to eight weeks), short visits.
   3. Examine thoroughly if new symptoms arise.
   4. Avoid unnecessary diagnostic procedures.
   5. Minimize medication use.
   6. Refer to psychiatrist or psychologist when appropriate but maintain ongoing relationship as primary therapeutic manager.

3. **The manipulating drug abuser**

Physician response: Anger.

Management tips:

1. Set limits and stick to them.
2. Never prescribe narcotics for someone else's patient.
3. Be suspicious of strange stories about lost pills.
4. Refer to pain clinic or detox program if patient is willing.

4. **The overly dependent patient**

Physician response: Gratification at first, then resentment.

Management tips:

1. Be wary of the patient with extreme gratitude.
2. Set firm limits for frequency of visits and calls.
3. Freely acknowledge to the patient your own human limitations.

5. **The terminally ill patient**

Physician response: Anger.

Management tips:

1. Realize that these patients are looking for care, not cure.
2. Avoid specific prognostic parameters.
3. Ensure that adequate comfort care measures are maintained.
4. Make an effort to be there for the patient.

6. **The noncompliant patient**

Physician response: Loss of control, then loss of interest.

Management tips:

1. Recognize limitations in changing patient's behavior.
2. Resist the desire to give up.
3. Change therapeutic plan to modalities that the patient will accept, realizing that you may have to settle for less than optimal treatment.

7. **The borderline personality**

   Physician response: Anger and hostility.

   Management tips:
   1. Refer for psychiatric co-care, but be aware of "splitting."
   2. Avoid drugs that are addictive.
   3. Set firm limits and be consistent.

SKILLS AND TECHNIQUES NEEDED TO MANAGE DIFFICULT PATIENTS

Physicians who are adept at managing difficult patients point out that when physicians avoid acknowledging such feelings, they are more likely to misdiagnose or mismanage a patient. Their recommendations include:

1. Stop disavowing intense or hateful feelings toward a patient.
2. Recognize that these feelings are, in a sense, part of the "diagnosis" for that particular patient. This concept must be used with caution — just because the physician is angry does not necessarily mean that the patient is manipulative.
3. Discuss feelings with colleagues in order to obtain their help.
4. Remember that, ultimately, it is not these feelings but how the physician behaves toward the patient that is most important.
5. Most patients need a stable, long-term relationship with a primary care physician who is not compelled to evaluate all symptoms extensively.

XI. PAIN MANAGEMENT/PALLIATIVE CARE

THE NEED FOR MORE AGGRESSIVE TREATMENT
Many patients and family members fear that pain control may be inadequate (with good reason). The prevalence of this fear may be responsible, in part, for the increasing interest in euthanasia and assisted death.

MISTAKES THAT ARE MADE
1. The drug selection may be poor. For example, meperidine (Demerol®) is clearly inferior to morphine for the control of the severe pain of bony metastases.
2. The dose may be inadequate or the dosing interval too long.
3. Physicians may fear causing addiction in patients who experience chronic pain or terminal illness and have to take large doses for long periods of time.
4. Physicians may prescribe inadequate doses of narcotics to patients who are terminally ill, for fear of inducing respiratory depression.

GOOD PAIN MANAGEMENT
1. **Choice/dose of drugs**
   Learn the appropriate drugs for given clinical situations and the proper dose and dosing interval.
2. **Knowledge about addiction**
   Addiction (true psychological dependence) is rare in patients who receive narcotics for pain, even if the drug must be continued for protracted periods. Tolerance — the need to increase the dose for the same pharmacologic effect — varies from patient to patient. Physiologic dependence occurs in all patients with long-term use, but opioids can be tapered over several days to avoid withdrawal symptoms.

3. **Respiratory depression**

Hospices and oncology services report that respiratory depression is uncommon in patients who are receiving opioids for the control of pain; if respiratory depression occurs, it is often from some cause other than the opioid. Pain itself is a respiratory stimulant, and the opioid effect on the respiratory center diminishes rapidly with chronic use. If the patient is terminally ill and the dose of opioid required to produce comfort does happen to depress respiration, it is still reasonable to allow the undesired effect (respiratory depression) in order to achieve the desired effect (relief of suffering) according to the recognized principle of double effect.

4. **Palliative sedation**

Physicians may have to resort to this procedure to relieve the suffering of a dying patient whose disease is incurable and whose symptoms are refractory (cannot be controlled despite aggressive efforts that do not compromise consciousness). Symptoms requiring deep sedation for relief include:

- Dyspnea (most common cause)
- Pain not controlled by opioid without distressing side-effects
- Agitated delirium, restlessness with myoclonus
- Unrelieved vomiting.

FURTHER READING

From Wanzer, et al.:

"In the patient whose dying process is irreversible, the balance between minimizing pain and suffering and potentially hastening death should be struck clearly in favor of pain relief. Narcotics and other pain medications should be given in whatever dose and by whatever route is necessary for relief. It is morally correct to increase the dose of narcotics to whatever dose is needed, even though the medication may contribute to the depression of respiration or blood pressure, the dulling of consciousness or even death, providing the primary goal of the physician is to relieve suffering. The proper dose of pain medication is the dose that is sufficient to relieve pain and suffering, even to the point of unconsciousness."

REFERENCES

Buchan ML, Tolle SW. Pain relief for dying persons: dealing with physicians' fears and concerns. *J Clin Ethics*. 1995;6:53-61.

Cherny NL, Portenoy RK. Sedation in the management of refractory symptoms: guidelines for evaluation and treatment. *J Palliative Care*. 1994;10:31-38.

Lo B, Rubenfeld G. Palliative sedation in dying patients: "we turn to it when everything else hasn't worked." *JAMA*. 2005;294(14):1810-1816.

Quill TE, Lo B, Brock DW. Palliative options of last resort. *JAMA*. 1997;278:2099-2104.

Rousseau P. Terminal sedation in the care of dying patients. *Arch Intern Med*. 1996;156:1785-1786.

Sulmasy DP, Pellegrino ED. The rule of double effect: clearing up the double talk. *Arch Intern Med*. 1999;159:545-550.

Wanzer SH, et al. The physician's responsibility toward hopelessly ill patients: a second look. *N Engl J Med*. 1989;320:844-849.

XII. AUTOPSY

NEED FOR AUTOPSIES

Physicians sometimes think autopsies are no longer necessary in this era of computed tomography and magnetic resonance imaging. Autopsies are still needed, however, for medical, legal, epidemiological, and familial reasons. The official in the relevant jurisdiction legally authorized to investigate deaths is known as the coroner. In many jurisdictions, that official may be required to be a pathologist or physician, and may be called a medical examiner.

INDICATIONS FOR AUTOPSY

1. Comply with medical examiner's (or coroner's) requirements
2. Clarify puzzling cases
3. Delineate suspected or unsuspected medical conditions
4. Provide useful information to the family
5. Reassure survivors with negative findings
6. Collect statistical data
7. Define environmental and occupational hazards
8. Provide legal and forensic information
9. Enhance clinical, pathological, and medical education.

MEDICAL EXAMINER (OR CORONER) CASES

These are cases that must, by law, be reported to the medical examiner:

1. Unexplained or unusual circumstances surrounding death
2. All homicides
3. All suicides
4. All deaths following abortion

5. All deaths due to poisoning (homicidal, suicidal, or accidental)
6. All deaths following accidents, regardless of whether the injury was the primary cause of death (for example, a patient hospitalized for treatment of fractures sustained in an automobile accident who dies in the hospital of a myocardial infarction still needs to be reported)
7. When no physician is in attendance
8. When the attending physician refuses to sign the death certificate.

If there is doubt about the need to report, it is best to call the medical examiner's or coroner's office.

NOTIFYING AND COUNSELING THE FAMILY

Immediately after pronouncing death:
1. Notify the attending physician and determine if he or she wishes to inform the family.
2. If the task is delegated to you, speak in person to the family, if possible. Phone only if necessary.
3. Identify yourself as the doctor caring for their loved one and let them know you have bad news to convey.
4. Inform them gently that their loved one has died, and avoid euphemisms such as "passed away" and "expired."
5. Express sympathy. Physical contact such as a hand on the shoulder may be appropriate.
6. If appropriate to the situation, you may wish to involve the hospital chaplain and/or the social worker.
7. Quietly and sensitively raise the question of autopsy, giving the reasons for its importance in this case (such as uncertainty of diagnosis, the family's need to know, scientific advancement).

8. Assure family that an open-casket funeral service is not precluded by the procedure, and — if you know this will be the case — that there is no cost to them.

OBTAINING CONSENT FOR AN AUTOPSY

Consent for the autopsy must be obtained in writing, by telegram, or by fax. Some states may allow phone consent with another hospital employee as "witness" on the line. Generally, consent should be obtained from the next of kin in the following order:
1. Surviving spouse. If none, then
2. Adult children. If none, then
3. Parents. If none, then
4. Brothers and sisters. If none, then
5. Any relative (or friend) who assumes custody of the body.
6. In some jurisdictions, if none of the above can be found within a specified period an autopsy may be performed without consent.

If the case is reported to the medical examiner and accepted for autopsy, family consent is not necessary; the family has no option for refusal. Furthermore, a consent signed by any agent listed above does not preclude an autopsy by the medical examiner.

AFTER THE DEATH (NO AUTOPSY DONE)

1. You may want to attend the funeral (if your relationship to the patient makes this appropriate).
2. Always send a card or a brief letter or make a follow-up call.
3. If possible, have the surviving caregiver return to the hospital for a follow-up conversation; this is a good time to resolve any questions or concerns.

AFTER THE DEATH (AUTOPSY DONE)

1. Same as above.
2. Your follow-up call should include information about the preliminary autopsy report. The pathologist who performed the autopsy may also be available for consultation.
3. Written autopsy reports are usually available within four to six weeks of the procedure. A copy can be given to the family personally or by letter.

XIII. ORGAN DONATION

SUITABLE DONORS
1. There is no age limit for solid organs or corneal donation. Organ procurement organizations (OPOs) evaluate donations on a case-by-case basis.
2. Donor must younger than 70 for bone and soft tissue donation.

TRANSPLANTABLE ORGANS
Kidney, liver, heart, lung, pancreas, and small bowel.

TRANSPLANTABLE TISSUES
Skin, long bone, heart valve, vein, tendon, and cornea.

CRITERIA FOR ORGAN DONATION
1. Solid organ donors must meet the criteria for brain death (section VII, page 28) and must be on ventilator support.
2. The issue of non-heart-beating cadaver donors (NHBCD) remains controversial but is current policy at some institutions. In patients for whom life-sustaining medical treatment withdrawal is ethically appropriate and who have indicated their wish to donate organs, the ventilator is discontinued with the expectation of imminent death. Hypotension, apnea, and cardiac arrest ensue, and the patient is pronounced dead by heart-lung death criteria. The withdrawal occurs in the operating room — or in close proximity — and the patient is taken quickly to the operating room. Organ procurement begins after a specified period (e.g., five minutes) after the declaration of death to assure the continued absence of cardiac and respiratory activity. This

protocol allows an additional pathway to organ donation besides those established by brain-death protocols. The controversy has arisen in part because of practitioners' comfort with the irreversibility of brain death, and the knowledge that cardiopulmonary arrest under some circumstances may be reversible. However, since in these circumstances death is expected and the intention is not to resuscitate the patient, when heart-lung death is declared, the patient is dead.

3. Bone and tissue donation occur within 24 hours of asystole.
4. Corneal donation occurs within four to six hours of asystole.
5. Patients with infection, sepsis, or malignancy are not candidates for organ donation.
6. These criteria are quite flexible; more organs and tissues from older donors are used now than in the past.

CONSENT FOR ORGAN DONATION

1. A signed donor card takes precedence over the wishes of any survivor. These wishes should be explained to the family.
2. The family of any potential donor (who does not have a specific contraindication to donation) must be asked about donation and should be encouraged to give permission (especially when the patient is brain dead and is thus a suitable donor for solid organs).
3. Even if the person did not sign a driver's license form for organ donation, the family may agree to donate organs.

COST OF ORGAN DONATION
Families need to be told that they are not responsible for any of the costs related to organ donation for transplant.

FUNERAL ARRANGEMENTS AFTER ORGAN DONATION
Assure the family that the body is released soon after the organs or tissues are removed and that funeral arrangements are rarely delayed. When donation is complete, prosthetic replacements are used to restore the body to its natural appearance. Open-casket viewing is possible with any type of donation.

INSTITUTIONAL RESOURCES
All institutions with transplant programs have someone with expertise in organ procurement who can give advice. A phone call to the coordinator on call is recommended before approaching the next of kin for permission.

REFERENCES

American Medical Association, Council on Ethical and Judicial Affairs. Ethical considerations in the allocation of organs and other scarce medical resources among patients. *Arch Intern Med.* 1995;155:29-40.

Ubel PA, Arnold RA, Caplan AL. Rationing failure: the ethical lessons of retransplantation of scarce vital organs. *JAMA.* 1993;270:2469-2474.

Youngner SJ, Arnold RM. Ethical, psychological, and public policy implications of procuring organs from non-heart beating cadaver donors. *JAMA.* 1993;269:2769-2774.

XIV. HIV/AIDS

Ethical dilemmas encountered in the care of patients with human immunodeficiency virus (HIV) and acquired immunodeficiency syndrome (AIDS) may include issues of compassion, medical futility, care of the incompetent patient, confidentiality, and management of the difficult patient (see also sections IV, V, IX, and X).

PHYSICIANS' RESPONSE TO THE RISK OF HIV/AIDS

Health professionals' fear of contracting AIDS will exist as long as there is a risk that HIV can be transmitted in the health-care setting. Despite infection-control procedures, a very small (much less than 1 percent) occupational risk exists. This risk requires a professional response: physicians have always had to set aside their personal fears to care for sick persons.

The physician may also have to overcome personal antipathies to patients of different cultural and socioeconomic backgrounds (such as intravenous-drug users) and different sexual orientations. If a gap exists between doctor and patient, ethical discussions regarding medical indications, the patient's preferences, allocation of resources, use of cardiopulmonary resuscitation (CPR), and treatment in the intensive care unit (ICU) are made more difficult.

The American Medical Association Council on Ethical and Judicial Affairs has stated, "A physician may not ethically refuse to treat a patient whose condition is within the physician's current realm of competence solely because the patient is seropositive. Persons who are seropositive should not be subjected to discrimination based on fear or prejudice," (*JAMA*. 1988; 259:1360-1361). Federal laws contain similar conditions.

Even though highly active antiretroviral treatment now prolongs the lives of many persons with HIV, the dilemmas faced in the early AIDS epidemic are still relevant. HIV remains one of the most serious and difficult to treat viral diseases. Perhaps physicians can learn from the response to HIV/AIDS to be better prepared to face the next serious epidemic.

RECOMMENDATIONS

1. Most patients with HIV infection benefit from combined drug therapy, which requires highly specialized clinical knowledge. For this reason, most HIV-positive patients are followed by infectious disease specialists.
2. In many cases, doctors must try to bridge the social or psychological gap between themselves and their patients.
3. New treatment regimens have decreased the morbidity and mortality of HIV infection, and it is now becoming more of a chronic rather than a terminal disease.
4. Sometimes, however, treatment becomes futile; the physician should then withdraw or withhold the treatment, using the skills and paradigms described in this text. Encouraging the patient to complete an advance directive helps decision making in these circumstances (see sections I, II, and XVII).

OTHER CONTAGIOUS DISEASES

Physicians may have responsibility for the care of patients with other contagious and potentially lethal diseases such as ebola, bird flu, and, perhaps, recurrence of plague or smallpox. The issues and ethical demands remain the same as in HIV/AIDS.

REFERENCES

American Medical Association, Council on Ethical and Judicial Affairs. Ethical issues involved in the growing AIDS crisis. *JAMA*. 1988;259:1360-1361.

Derse AR. HIV and AIDS: legal and ethical issues in the emergency department. *Emerg Med Clin North Am*. 1995;13:213-223.

Verghese A. *My Own Country: A Doctor's Story of a Town and Its People in the Age of AIDS*. New York: Simon and Schuster; 1994.

Wachter RM, Luce JM, Hopewell PC. Critical care of patients with AIDS. *JAMA*. 1992;267:541-547.

Zuger A, Miles SH. Physicians, AIDS, and occupational risk: historic traditions and ethical obligations. *JAMA*. 1987;258:1924-1928.

XV. PEDIATRIC ISSUES

STANDARDS: BEST INTEREST VERSUS SUBSTITUTED JUDGMENT

One of the most difficult aspects of making decisions regarding the treatment of children is knowing what is in the best interest of the child. Nonetheless, this is the appropriate standard for decision making. Parents should be involved in this process. The substituted-judgment standard cannot generally be employed in cases involving children because, unlike adults, pediatric patients have never possessed decision-making capacity. The wishes of older children should be considered in decision making, and some children who are "mature minors" (see section IV, page 21) can be treated like adults.

THE PEDIATRICIAN AS CHILD ADVOCATE

The primary role of the attending pediatrician is that of child advocate. Reasonable medical measures that are in the best interest of the child should be employed, with at least a trial of treatment even in the most critically ill children. As in adult medicine, futility may be a contraindication to continued treatment in some cases.

Pediatricians have encouraged immunization, Head Start, nutrition programs, and other innovative initiatives to improve the lives of children. Pediatricians have clearly demonstrated that adequate food and housing, proper sanitation, and childhood immunizations are more potent overall lifesavers than technical medical interventions.

ADVISING PARENTS

As advisors to the parents of their patients, pediatricians can counsel and support them as they reach decisions regarding the best interest of their child.

This is a difficult process, for the physician must be as objective as possible in giving an opinion or medical recommendation. The pediatrician may fail in the role of advisor in two ways. He or she may hide behind the "objectivity" of the medical facts and refuse to give any guidance on what is medically and ethically correct, merely saying "These are the options. What do you want me to do?" Conversely, the physician may knowingly or unknowingly manipulate parents into making a decision the physician prefers by relating only those facts that would support that particular decision.

It is useful to give the parents time and to encourage them to get a second or even a third opinion in difficult circumstances. If the ethical issues remain unclear, a consultation with the ethics committee may be appropriate.

NEONATAL INTENSIVE CARE

In the past, medical care for critically ill newborns was mainly supportive. Data collected in the neonatal intensive care unit (NICU) confirm that gains have been made in the survival of infants with increasingly low birth weights. The limit for providing ventilatory support in the 1960s was 1,500 grams; 40 years later, the limit was 400 grams.

The success, however, is not unqualified. Ventilatory management has been difficult, and multiple complications may occur. The low-birth-weight neonate may have patent ductus arteriosus, immature brain and germinal matrix, and incomplete retinal vascularization. Increased attention to and funding of neonatal intensive care technology may be diverting attention and funding from basic prenatal care. As is true in adult medicine, the recent focus on high technology is threatening the traditional primary care focus of pediatrics.

ETHICAL ISSUES

Neonatal ethical issues focus on the aggressiveness of treatment and resuscitation of infants who are already being treated aggressively in the NICU. Pediatric ethics issues for the mature minor mirror those of the adult patient. The capacity of children to be involved in decisions depends upon their age and intellectual capacity.

REFERENCES

Lantos JD, et al. Providing and forgoing resuscitative therapy for babies of very low birth weight. *J Clin Ethics*. 1992;3:283-287.

Neonatal resuscitation guidelines. *Circulation*. 2005;112:IV-188-IV-195.

President's Commission for the Study of Ethical Problems in Medicine and Biomedical and Behavioral Research. *Deciding to Forego Life-Sustaining Treatment*. Washington, DC: US Government Printing Office; 1983.

XVI. CONFLICT OF INTEREST

The earliest ethical treatises prohibited physicians from splitting fees with those who referred them patients. Jonsen (1983) noted that the profession's main dilemma is balancing altruism and greed.

1. Physicians should avoid arrangements that benefit them only by decreasing the quality of care (for example, incentives which favor many unnecessary procedures in fee-for-service practice or wholly inadequate numbers of needed procedures in managed-care practice).

2. While dual loyalties are inevitable, physicians should err on the patient's side. For example, hospitals often want to decrease the length of stay, even though optimum care for some patients requires an increased length of stay. Most institutions and insurance companies rightfully expect physicians to be advocates for patients based on best medical interests. Without such advocacy, valuable checks and balances against corporate greed are lost.

3. Physicians may ethically own their own offices, labs, and medical equipment without an inherent conflict of interest. This historical practice seems to have stood the test of time and is convenient for patients and doctors alike — but the use must not be abused.

4. Physicians should avoid owning unique medical devices or facilities that generate profitable self-referral. After all, that concept is really fee-splitting through use of a scarce technology.

5. Physicians should not accept large gifts, trips, or favors from pharmaceutical companies — (accept nothing that you would not like reported in the local newspaper).

6. Physicians should not be involved in the process of "bedside rationing." The only responsibility of the ethical physician is

to be an advocate for the patient. If distribution is to be fair and just, rationing decisions must be made by society so that any limits the physician imposes on patients are shared by all physicians and patients in the same clinical setting.

FURTHER READING

The patient-physician covenant

The following statement was written by a group of medical ethicists and endorsed by the American College of Physicians and the American Board of Internal Medicine:

"Medicine is, at its center, a moral enterprise grounded in a covenant of trust. This covenant obliges physicians to be competent and to use their competence in the patient's best interests. Physicians, therefore, are both intellectually and morally obliged to act as advocates for the sick wherever their welfare is threatened and for their health at all times. Today, this covenant of trust is significantly threatened. From within, there is growing legitimation of the physician's materialistic self interest; from without, for-profit forces press the physician into the role of commercial agent to enhance the profitability of health care organizations. Such distortions of the physician's responsibility degrade the physician-patient relationship that is the central element and structure of clinical care.

To capitulate to these alterations of the trust relationship is to significantly alter the physician's role as healer, caregiver, helper, and advocate for the sick and for the health of all.

By its traditions and its very nature, medicine is a special kind of human activity — one that cannot be pursued effectively without the virtues of humility, honesty, intellectual integrity, compassion, and effacement of excessive self interest. These traits mark physicians as members of a moral community dedicated to something other than its own self interest.

Our first obligation must be to serve the good of those persons who seek our help and trust us to provide it. Physicians, as physicians, are not, and must never be, commercial entrepreneurs, gate closers, or agents of fiscal policy that runs counter to our trust. Any defection from primacy of the patient's well-being places the patient at risk by treatment that may compromise quality of or access to medical care.

We believe the medical profession must reaffirm the primacy of its obligation to the patient through national, state, and local professional societies; our academic, research, and hospital organizations; and especially through personal behavior. As advocates for the promotion of health and support for the sick, we are called upon to discuss, defend, and promulgate medical care by every ethical means available. Only by caring and advocating for the patient can the integrity of the profession be affirmed. Thus we honor our covenant of trust with patients."

Reprinted with permission from Crawshaw R, et al. The patient-physician covenant. *JAMA*. 1995;273:1553.

REFERENCES

Jecker, NS, Jonsen, AR. Healthcare as a commons. *Cambridge Q*. 1995;4:207-216.

Jonsen, AR. Watching the doctor. *N Engl J Med*. 1983;308(25):1531-1535.

XVII. ADVANCE DIRECTIVES

DEFINITION
An advance directive (AD) is a statement a patient makes, while still in possession of decision-making capacity, about how treatment decisions should be made at some future time if he or she loses the capacity to make such decisions.

TYPES OF AD
1. Living will (LW) statutory form
2. Power of attorney for healthcare (PAHC) statutory form
3. Nonstatutory forms

LIVING WILL
1. **Provisions**

   Most statutory forms are documents stating the desire to die a "natural" death and not to be kept alive by medical treatment and machines. In many states, the principal may also stipulate that fluid and nutrition are to be discontinued in the event of persistent vegetative state (PVS).

2. **Activation**

   Usually the LW becomes effective on the determination of "terminal" illness or "imminent" death (death expected within six months) or, in some jurisdictions, the diagnosis of PVS made by two physicians.

POWER OF ATTORNEY FOR HEALTHCARE
1. **Provisions**

   Most statutory forms provide a way for the principal to appoint a person to act as healthcare agent (who may also be known as a proxy or surrogate) to make healthcare decisions in the event that the principal loses the capacity to make decisions. The PAHC allows the principal to add specific directions, and often the agent may be given authority to have feeding tubes withheld or withdrawn.

2. **Activation**

The PAHC becomes effective when two physicians, or one physician and one psychologist, determine that the principal is no longer decisional.

PREFERENCE

Patients may ask for the physician's advice about ADs. The statutory form of the PAHC is the best choice because it allows all of the options of a LW and has the added advantage of providing an agent — someone who knows the principal well and can take an active role in the decision-making process on the patient's behalf. The PAHC also allows for the addition of specific instructions to the agent. There is no advantage to filling out both forms.

Note: The laws regarding LWs and PAHCs vary from state to state. It is wise to check the provisions and standards for activation in your own jurisdiction.

FURTHER READING

Living will
  Strengths
  • Allows the physician to understand the patient's wishes and motivations.
  • Extends the patient's autonomy, self-control, and self-determination.
  • Relieves the patient's anxiety about unwanted treatment.
  • Relieves physician's anxiety about legal liability.
  • Reduces family strife and sense of guilt.
  • Improves communication and trust between patient and physician.

Weaknesses
- Applicable only to those in PVS or the terminally ill (patients who have a disease that is incurable and will die regardless of treatment).
- Death must be imminent (likely to occur within six months).
- Ambiguous terms may be difficult to later interpret.
- There is no proxy decision maker, so:
  - It requires prediction of final illness scenario and available treatment.
  - It requires physician to make decisions on the basis of an interpretation of a document.

Note: In light of these weaknesses, it is strongly recommended that patients complete the PAHC and not the LW. There is no advantage to having both.

Power of attorney for healthcare (PAHC)
Activation of PAHC
Lack of decision-making capacity must be certified by two physicians or one physician and a psychologist who have examined the patient. Until then, the patient makes all the decisions.
Advantages
- Physician has someone to talk with — a proxy, a knowledgeable surrogate — who can provide a substituted judgment of how the patient would have chosen. If the agent is unable to provide a substituted judgment, the agent and physician together can use the best-interest standard (how a reasonable person might choose in consideration of the benefit-burden concept of proportionality).
- Provides flexibility; this decreases ambiguity and uncertainty because there is no way to predict all possible scenarios.
- Authority of agent can be limited as person desires.
- Avoids family conflict about rightful agent.
- Provides legal immunity for physicians who follow dictates.
- Allows appointment of a nonrelative (especially valuable for persons who may be alienated from their families).
- Most forms can be completed without an attorney.
- Principal may add specific instructions to the agent such as the following:

I value a full life more than a long life. If my suffering is intense and irreversible, or if I have lost the ability to interact with others and have no reasonable hope of regaining this ability even though I have no terminal illness, I do not want to have my life prolonged. I would then ask not to be subjected to surgery or to resuscitation procedures, or to intensive care services or to other life-prolonging measures, including the administration of antibiotics or blood products or artificial nutrition and hydration (adapted from Bok, 1996).

Nonstatutory forms

These are forms that are not codified in state law. They may contain ambiguous language, which can cause difficulty in interpretation. In many states, nonstatutory forms — unlike the statutory forms of the LW and PAHC — may not provide legal immunity for physicians who follow the dictates of the document.

Patient Self-Determination Act (PSDA)

This federal law, which went into effect in 1991, involves all Medicare and Medicaid providers (hospitals, nursing homes, hospices, and health-maintenance organizations). According to the provisions of the Patient Self-Determination Act (PSDA), all healthcare providers must:

1. Give all patients written information at the time of admission, advising them of their rights to refuse any treatments and to have an AD. This is usually done by nursing or social service staff shortly after admission, but patients may ask physicians about ADs.
2. Document the presence of an AD in the patient's record.
3. Have written policies respecting the rights of patients to have an AD and to refuse treatment.
4. Make provisions to educate staff and community on these issues.
5. Prohibit discrimination against a person because they do or do not have an AD.

Some misconceptions patients have about ADs

1. **"If I sign one, I can't change my mind."**

    An AD can easily be revoked — orally, in writing, or by filling out a new AD that supersedes the old.

2. **"I'm young and/or I'm in good health, so I don't need an AD."**
    The *Cruzan* and *Quinlan* cases — two prominent court cases that drew attention of the public to this issue — involved women in their twenties.

3. **"If I have an AD, paramedics won't resuscitate me."**
    Because the standard of activation for the LW is the presence of a terminal condition and for the PAHC is loss of decision-making capacity, these documents, as a rule, do not speak to emergency situations; insufficient time exists to determine the presence of the effective activating elements. An occasional exception is the chronically ill individual who specifies do not resuscitate in the PAHC.

4. **"My family might not want me to sign an AD."**
    Families generally welcome the opportunity to discuss these issues, and the presence of an AD can do much to relieve family guilt if it becomes necessary to withdraw or withhold treatment.

5. **"My spouse/family knows what I want" or "My physician knows what I want."**
    Numerous surveys report that neither family members nor physicians are accurate in their estimation of patients' preferences; designation of an agent with specific instructions is the best way to circumvent this problem.

Some misconceptions physicians have about ADs

1. **"The provisions of the AD may require me to act counter to my philosophy and conscience."**
    The physician needs to discuss the AD with the patient to make sure that no conflict exists between the patient's desires and the physician's principles. If a conflict is present, it may be necessary to transfer the patient to the care of another physician.

2. **"I know what my patients want."**
    See item 5 above.

3. **"I can't bill for the time spent discussing these ADs."**
    This is an important obligation, regardless of the financial reward. However, the service can usually be billed under the codes for counseling, patient education, and preventive care.

Recommendations to patients and the public regarding ADs

1. Think about the issues and your specific wishes; discuss them with family.
2. Complete the PAHC form rather than the LW form.
3. Discuss your desires fully with both the primary and alternate agents. You may want to add some written instructions.
4. Discuss the decisions with your personal physician to get agreement on specifics.
5. These documents need to be circulated widely. Copies of the documents should be given to primary and alternate agents, close family members, personal physician, and personal attorney.

Recommendations to physicians

1. It is the physician's responsibility to initiate discussion with all decisional patients, regardless of age. This is best done in the office (clinic) at a nonthreatening time. Use of printed informational material is helpful, as is the availability of PAHC forms in the office.
2. Describe the settings in which an AD is important. Tell patients that you, as their physician, will be in a better position to direct their treatment with a written AD.
3. Assure patients that symptomatic care and treatment will never be withheld.
4. Patients may need time to reflect and discuss these issues with their families. It may be a good idea to initiate the topic at one clinic visit and to discuss it further at a later visit.
5. Document a patient's oral statements if an AD is not completed. If an AD is completed, file it in the patient's record.
6. Review the AD with the patient to prevent misunderstandings.
7. Emphasize the need for the patient to discuss the AD fully with his or her family.
8. Complete an AD (PAHC) yourself.

REFERENCES

Bok S. Personal directions for care at the end of life. *N Engl J Med.* 1976;295: 362-369.

Lynn J, et al. Perceptions by family members of the dying experience of older and seriously ill patients. *Ann Intern Med.* 1997;126:97-106.

Miles SH, Koepp R, Weber EP. Advance end-of-life treatment planning. *Arch Intern Med.* 1996;156:1062-1068.

Pearlman RA, Uhlmann RF, Jecker NS. Spousal understanding of patient quality of life: implications for surrogate decisions. *J Clin Ethics.* 1992;3:114-120.

XVIII. ETHICS CONSULTATION

ETHICS COMMITTEES

Institutional ethics committees (ECs) have many different con-figurations. Many are standing committees of the medical staff, which report to the medical executive committee or governing staff of the hospital. Most meet monthly, or more frequently as occasion demands. Typically ECs have three tasks:

1. Education — of committee members, staff, and the com-munity
2. Policy formulation — the EC is not a policy-making body but will suggest policy on request of the medical staff or hospital administration
3. Case consultation — on request.

REASONS FOR CASE CONSULTATION

An ethics consultation might be considered for some of the following reasons:

1. For clarification of issues regarding decision-making ca-pacity, informed consent, or advance directives
2. To provide recommendations for cases involving do-not-resuscitate orders or withdrawal of treatment
3. To help in resolution of ethical conflict — between family and caregivers, patient and caregivers, patient and family, or among staff members.

FURTHER READING

Case consultation method

(This is the approach used by the authors' institutional EC.)

1. Response to consultation request

The consultant or the EC member who initially responds to the re-quest for consultation should consider the following:

- Who requested the consult? If it was not the attending physician, does he or she agree?
- What is the ethical problem? Is the problem ethical — or does it involve legal, social, or psychological issues; staff conflict; or miscommunication? Is it a problem that needs referral to another service?
- What specifically is being requested of the EC? Clarification of the problem? Mediation? Recommendations?

2. Evaluation by the responding consultant
- See the patient. If the patient has decision-making capacity, notify him or her of the nature of the visit.
- Interview nursing personnel, other personnel, and family members.
- Discuss the problem with the attending physician and other consultants.
- Review the chart.

3. Decision about emergency meeting of full EC
- If the problem is uncomplicated, common, and the reaction of the EC can be anticipated, the consultant may resolve it.
- If the problem is unusual, problematic, delicate, or has legal ramifications, a full emergency EC meeting is called.

Assessment of the ethical problem
(By either the initial consultant or the entire EC)

1. Medical facts
- Decision-making capacity of the patient
- Current medical status, diagnosis, and prognosis
- Recommended treatment and reasonable alternative treatments
- Effect of no treatment
- Assessment of the patient's life expectancy
- Views of caregivers

2. Patient's preference
- Has the patient been informed and given time to reflect on options?
- What are the patient's personal/social factors? What is his or her value system?

- • What is the patient's personal assessment of quality of life?
- • What are the patient's current expressed choices?
- • Are there any advance directives?

3. External factors
- • Family
  - • How well do they know and represent the patient?
  - • Do they understand the situation? Are they in agreement?
  - • Is there any conflict of interest?
  - • If there is no advance directive, who is the decision maker?
- • Religion — are religious or cultural values involved?
- • Expense — is it a factor in the patient's decisions?
- • Legal issues
  - • Are there applicable hospital policies or state statutes?
  - • Is there potential liability?

Problem resolution
1. Make sure the information is complete.
2. Delineate the ethical problem clearly.
3. Clarify the options.
   - • Did we assure as much patient autonomy as possible?
   - • Are our recommendations consistent with the patient's preferences or best interest?
   - • Are our recommendations consistent with ethical principles?

Reporting
1. Recommendations are made as recommendations. It is up to the attending physician to take or reject them, as is true of all consultations.
2. Report of the consultation will be placed on the chart, unless requested otherwise.
3. Full report of the consultation will be detailed in the minutes of the EC for educational and quality purposes, but special care will be taken to preserve patient confidentiality.
4. Full minutes as required by medical staff bylaws will go to the medical staff executive committee.

Follow Up

In many situations, the consultant will need to follow the patient in order to be available for further consultation. The consultant should also check on the patient's status and make progress reports to the EC for educational purposes.

REFERENCES

Fletcher JC, Siegler M. What are the goals of ethics consultation? a consensus statement. *J Clin Ethics.* 1996;7:122-126.

La Puma J, Schiedermayer D. *Ethics Consultation: A Practical Guide.* Boston: Jones and Bartlett; 1994.

Walker MU. Keeping moral spaces open: new images of ethics consulting. *Hastings Cent Rep.* 1993;23:33-40.

XIX. EUTHANASIA AND PHYSICIAN-ASSISTED DEATH

DEFINITIONS
1. Euthanasia
The physician participates in an intentional, deliberate act to cause the immediate death of a person with terminal, incurable, or painful disease by the medical administration of a lethal drug.

2. Physician-assisted death (also known as physician-assisted suicide)
The physician provides the lethal drug with instructions for its use but is not the agent. The patient decides when and if to use the drug. Most, but not all, ethicists agree that euthanasia and physician-assisted death differ from one another significantly because of the agency. In euthanasia the physician is the direct agent; in physician-assisted death it is the patient who is the direct agent.

LEGAL ASPECTS
Euthanasia is illegal in all states. Suicide is not illegal, but all states except Oregon now have some sort of legal prohibition against assisted suicide. In the other states there is a specific law against assisting a suicide, or prosecution is possible under other existing statutes.

ETHICAL ASPECTS
1. American Medical Association Policy
"The intentional termination of the life of one human being by another is contrary to public policy, medical tradition, and the most fundamental measures of human value and worth" (AMA. *Euthanasia*).

2. American College of Physicians Ethics Manual

"Although a patient may refuse a medical intervention and the physician may comply with this refusal, the physician must never intentionally and directly cause death or assist a patient to commit suicide" (*Ann Intern Med.* 1989;111: 245-335).

STATE INITIATIVES

Initiatives placed before the people of Washington in 1991 and California in 1992 to allow physician-assisted death failed in both states by relatively close margins. A ballot measure in Oregon to allow physician assistance in suicide for suffering patients with terminal illness passed in 1994. It was never implemented because of legal challenge. Oregon voters in 1997 reaffirmed support (favored by 60 percent), and the federal appeals court lifted the injunction. Thus, Oregon is the only state in which physician-assisted death (but not euthanasia) is legal.

Federal appeals court decisions in California and New York that upheld the lower court decision that declared the state statutes against assisted suicide unconstitutional were appealed to the U.S. Supreme Court. The Court considered both decisions together and rendered a unanimous decision that the state statutes against assisted suicide did not violate either the "due process" or equal protection provisions of the 14th Amendment of the U.S. Constitution. Thus, the two federal court decisions were negated. The opinions of several Supreme Court justices affirm the following:

1. The right of competent patients to discontinue or to withhold any treatment, even that considered life-sustaining
2. The right of competent patients to receive sufficient medication to relieve pain, even if that dose causes shortening of the patient's life

3. The right of competent patients whose suffering cannot otherwise be relieved to have terminal sedation
4. Because none of the above actions are considered suicide, physicians who accede to such patient requests cannot be considered to be "assisting a suicide."

The Court also allowed that the issue is not settled and that individual state legislatures might in the future take action legitimizing assisted suicide. Further attempts have followed. The Oregon experience has shown that the small number of patients (less than 0.1 percent of deaths) who choose this option do so not because of pain, but because of loss of autonomy, loss of enjoyment of activities, and loss of bodily function. Because this issue will not go away, physicians as a group need to consider thoughtfully the professional response to this situation.

THE PHYSICIAN'S RESPONSE

It is the responsibility of caring physicians to analyze the stimuli for these initiatives that have such widespread public support and to attempt to change those factors that are amenable to change. Prominent public fears that fuel this debate:
1. The concern that the pain experienced by a terminally ill patient will not be controlled adequately
2. The worry about loss of control and the indignity of dependence during the final illness
3. The concern that medical technology will continue to be used inappropriately, thus delaying an "easy" death.

By providing adequate pain control to terminally ill patients without fearing addiction or respiratory depression, physicians will help assuage the first concern. Use of appropriate palliative measures and increased reliance on hospice care will relieve many of the other concerns. By strongly recommending the use of advance directives and discussing these issues with their patients, physicians can reduce the burden of end-of-life decision making. If all of these interventions are carried out successfully, the stimulus for state initiatives should decrease. However, regardless of the effectiveness of good pain control and palliative care, there will remain a small but significant group of patients for whom no alternative to death is acceptable and for whom aid in dying is not irrational. Each physician will have to decide what the appropriate response should be.

REFERENCES

American College of Physicians. Ethics manual, part I: history; the patient: other physicians. *Ann Intern Med.* 1989;111:245-335.

American Medical Association, Council on Ethical and Judicial Affairs. Decisions near the end of life. *JAMA.* 1992;267:2229-2233.

American Medical Association, Council on Ethical and Judicial Affairs, *Euthanasia.* Chicago: American Medical Association; June 1988. Report 12:1-40.

Brody H. Assisted death: a compassionate response to a medical failure. *N Engl J Med.* 1992;327:1384-1388.

Miller FC. A communitarian approach to physician-assisted death. *Cambridge Q.* 1997;6:78-87.

Quill TE, Cassel CK, Meier DE. Care of the hopelessly ill: proposed clinical criteria for physician-assisted suicide. *N Engl J Med.* 1992;327:1380-1383.

Quill TE, Lo B, Brock DW. Palliative options of last resort: a comparison of voluntarily stopping eating and drinking, terminal sedation, physician-assisted suicide, and voluntary active euthanasia. *JAMA.* 1997;278:2099-2104.

XX. ABORTION

Much of the argument concerns beliefs regarding the time of onset of life. Some consider the onset of life to occur at the time of conception. Some believe that ensoulment occurs at the time of the union of sperm and ovum; from that time on, through the embryo phase and fetal development, the new individual has all the rights of personhood, so that any interference in development is tantamount to murder. Other traditions maintain that personhood comes only after the child is born. Still others believe that no rights accrue to an embryo, but that the developing fetus has increasing rights dependent upon progress toward the ability to exist outside of the womb.

In the 1973 U.S. Supreme Court decision (*Roe v. Wade*) the Court did not attempt to answer the question of when personhood begins, but instead balanced the rights of the state against the rights of the mother in a trimester-based analysis. The court held that in the first trimester, the state cannot restrict the right of the mother to an abortion. In the second trimester, the state may regulate abortion to protect maternal health. During the third trimester, when the fetus is viable, the state may regulate or prohibit abortion except as necessary to protect the life or health of the mother.

Scientific evidence about the inner life of the fetus is evolving. Neuronal connections in the brain and demonstrable brain waves cannot be identified in the fetus until about the beginning of the third trimester. Lung development sufficient to allow breathing does not happen until about the end of the second trimester.

Particular difficulty lies in the decision to abort a fetus found to have severe abnormalities incompatible with life (e.g., anencephaly). This discovery often occurs after the first trimester, so a late abortion may need to be considered. In contemplation of abortion after the second trimester (rarely necessary), the life or health of the mother is an important factor in this difficult decision-making process.

In a pluralistic society that is deeply divided over this issue, the debate continues in the legislative and judicial arenas. Physicians come to this issue from many different backgrounds and bring their own emotions and convictions. Physicians and other health-care practitioners should be able to refuse to participate in procedures that they deem immoral without compromising the ability of the patient to seek care from another practitioner. It is important that physicians treat patients (and other practitioners) respectfully when their views differ on this unresolved ethical issue.

FURTHER READING

Opinion of Justice Harry Blackmun in *Roe v. Wade*:
"We forthwith acknowledge our awareness of the sensitive and emotional nature of the abortion controversy, of the vigorous opposing views, even among physicians, and of the deep and seemingly absolute convictions that the subject inspires. One's philosophy, one's experience, one's exposure to the raw edges of human existence, one's religious training, one's attitude toward life and family and their values, and the moral standards one establishes and seeks to observe, are all likely to influence and color one's thinking and conclusions about abortion."

REFERENCE

Roe v. Wade, 410 U.S. 113 (1973).

XXI. THE PHYSICIAN'S PROFESSIONAL RESPONSIBILITIES

THE FUNDAMENTAL GOALS OF MEDICINE

The general goals of medicine include the following:

1. Prevention of disease and untimely death
2. Cure of disease, when possible
3. Improvement or maintenance of functional status when cure is not possible
4. Palliation (relief of pain and suffering), pursuit of a peaceful death, and comfort care in all situations
5. Patient education and counseling

Good clinical judgment requires a realistic understanding of the goals of treatment in a particular case. Physician and patient together should determine which goals are actually possible. Often a doctor and patient can agree that the goal should be palliation and comfort. Unfortunately, both physician and patient often fail to acknowledge the need to change goals when cure becomes impossible.

THE DOCTOR'S DUTIES

The central responsibility of the clinician is to use his or her technical expertise to respond to a patient's request for help by:

1. Making an accurate diagnosis of the patient's condition
2. Informing and educating the patient about the diagnosis
3. Recommending the course of action the clinician considers to be best
4. Discussing the benefits and risks of this course and of reasonable treatment alternatives
5. Discussing prognosis if treated or untreated

6. Carrying out with technical skill the necessary diagnostic and therapeutic procedures
7. Assuring the patient that he or she will not be abandoned.

INDIVIDUALIZING TREATMENT
In making a recommendation about clinical care, physicians need to evaluate the individual patient in terms of
1. The patient's comprehension and self-understanding
2. The organic seriousness of the condition
3. The seriousness of the condition in the patient's eyes
4. The need for urgent action
5. The physical, psychological, and social impact of the options on the patient
6. The ability of the patient to participate in his or her own care
7. The patient's values, beliefs, fears, and hopes.

MORAL DECISION MAKING
Clinicians are responsible for reaching a decision that is not only clinically and technically sound but is also morally appropriate and suitable for the specific problems of the particular patient being treated. The medical (technical) aspects of the decision answer the question, "What *can* be done for this patient?" The moral component involves the patient's wishes and answers the question, "What *ought* to be done for this patient?"

REWARDS
Quill and Cassel summarize the rewards of medicine:
"Clinical medicine is ultimately a humbling and exhilarating profession, filled with joy, sorrow, and an overabundance of uncertainty that comes with establishing a genuine long-term connection with patients. To practice medicine with a commit-

ment to caring and to be there no matter what the future holds is to experience the richness of the human condition over and over again and to know one has made a difference" (*Ann Intern Med.* 1995;122:373).

REFERENCES

Groopman, J. *How Doctors Think.* New York: Houghton, Mifflin Co; 2007.

McCullough LB. John Gregory (1724-1773) and the invention of professional relationships in medicine. *J Clin Ethics.* 1997;8:11-21.

Peabody FW. The care of the patient. *JAMA.* 1927;88:877-882.

Quill TE, Cassel CK. Non-abandonment: a central obligation for physicians. *Ann Intern Med.* 1995;122:368-374.

Specifying the goals of medicine. *Hastings Cent Rep.* November-December 1996;26(special supplement):9-16.

CPSIA information can be obtained at www.ICGtesting.com
Printed in the USA
BVOW04s2134170713

326129BV00008B/208/P

9 781555 720612